Searching For Daylight

I0117211

Kathryn Shaw

chipmunkapublishing
the mental health publisher

Kathryn Shaw

Published by
Chipmunkapublishing
PO Box 6872
Brentwood
Essex CM13 1ZT
United Kingdom

http://www.chipmunkapublishing.com

Chipmunkapublishing gratefully acknowledge the support of Arts Council England.

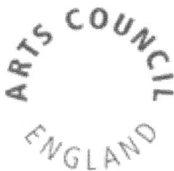

PART 1

1984 – 1985

Aged 14 – 15

Kathryn Shaw

Searching For Daylight

6th September 1984 – 23:17

Life's Mountain

Trudging through life is like climbing a mountain,
Out of reach so far up is the top.
The harder you climb, the harder it seems
And you are more likely to drop.

On your long journey, rocks bar your way,
The path can get rugged and rough
And however carefully you may tread,
You just can't be careful enough.

Sometimes you may think you've reached the peak
And all around you is light.
Then you look up, see a higher path
And the day quickly blackens to night.

You may lose your way through the wandering
paths,
Your mind gets confused with the fear,
And just when you feel that you cannot go on,
A new stronger path may appear.

So what is the point of climbing this mountain,
You know you cannot reach the top.
I think the fear that makes you keep climbing,
Is not knowing what's there when you stop.

So everyone climbs there own mountain,
In search of their hidden dreams.
And the dingy dull path that they follow,
Goes on forever it seems.

Kathryn Shaw

14th September 1984 – 23:40

Lost

Lost and alone like a solitary bubble,
Floating through miles of endless grey sky.
Not knowing your place or destination,
Just drifting along as the winds softly sigh.

Clouds gather above and rain pours downwards,
Filling your mind with the mists of despair.
Thoughts become jumbled, feelings are hidden,
Lost in damp-darkness of storm-heavy air.

Your life is just one of many around you,
Swept away by the wind and lost in the rain.
So what is the point, why should you keep trying?
You can't help but lose when there's nothing to gain.

Searching For Daylight

9th October 1984 – 23:48

Clouds

Why, when my life is going just right,
Do familiar black clouds block my way?
Why, when I try to talk to a friend,
Does my mind never know what to say?
I don't know where the answers have fled,
Lost, hidden far out of my sight.
I never know where to start searching,
When closing in softly, is night.
Before today my life seemed just fine,
The clouds had all lifted away.
I left my old feelings behind me,
But, of course, that was yesterday.
Now the sun is yet again hidden,
The dark mists inside block my view.
My mind is closed in, in darkness,
Still awaiting the soft touch of dew.
More cobwebs close in to destroy me.
My thoughts are destroyed by their spread.
The worst hate you ever could think of,
Glistens and winks on each thread.
Invisible clouds rain above me,
Visible tears fill my eyes,
As way deep down inside me,
A cold gale moans and cries.

28th October 1984 – 21:33

Shadows

Visions drifting, reality closing,
Filling dreams once filled with hope.
Life goes on, but death can linger,
Always hidden, watching, waiting.

"Life is but a passing shadow",
Many shadows hide the sun.
The sun can't win so why keep trying.
What's the point, so why go on.

Searching For Daylight

12th November 1984 – 22:51

Nothing

Feelings bottled up, strangled inside,
Jumbled and confused, trying to get free,
Blocking passages to freedom, hiding the keys,
Mixed up, covering happy thoughts.

Tears dry, unable to flow,
From already aching eyes.
Frustration fills the mind, slowly killing,
Dampening, obscuring, blackening.

Life becomes a floating dream,
Slowly passing by, drifting away,
And it doesn't seem to really matter,
Because nothing does any more.

The dream becomes a nightmare,
Full of darkened shapes and colours,
Visions of terror and hatred,
Appearing, looming up, and then gone.

The point, the aim, have all gone.
Nothing left but an empty vision,
Of what life used to be,
Before this…

Kathryn Shaw

13th November 1984 – 23:32

Hell

Men sweat and work forever,
Clanking of chains, roaring of fires.
Piercing screams fill the air,
The stench of sweat and heat is everywhere.

Perspiration gleams on every limb,
But the people cannot stop, though exhausted by
the heat.
They toil on, tired, nearly dropping, but cannot stop.
Serpents hiss and glide among their feet,

Making, no forcing, the work to go on.
Damp sweat drips from the walls,
Running, oozing to form streams on the floor.
This is no place to be:

It's a place where sins are repaid a thousand times,
And lost in the sweat, heat and screams of the air.
For this is somewhere no one wants to go,
A place filled and overflowing with death,

A place ruled by the devil,
A place called Hell.

Searching For Daylight

13th November 1984 – 23:50

Depression

It closes in steadily,
Towering over, blackening out,
Until the last chink of light,
Flees from the throbbing mind.
Then, slowly at first,
The mind begins to decay and rot,
The once bright thoughts turn dark and damp and dead.
Cobwebs form in corners,
Floods of tears wash through,
Filling the mind with dread
Of what the future has to hold.
Then it settles, like damp, cold snow
In the depths of the mind.
It works, destroying like the devil,
In the depths of hell.
It forces sadness and destroys all hope.
It fights as hate and kills the love.
It's the devil's clouds come to rest,
In the mind, as depression.

15th November 1984 – 20:42

Hate

Hate confuses the depths of any mind,
Killing, twisting, mixing emotions.
Turning the mind into a stormy mass
Of torrents of rushing thoughts.

Thinking normally becomes impossible,
Visions and dreams become reality,
That doesn't seem to be real,
Just a picture floating in a washed out mind.

Life becomes impossible to live,
With hate uppermost in the mind,
Covering all other happy thoughts
In a blanket of innocent fear.

Hate is impossible to overcome,
It just lies, waiting, resting,
Ready to kill once more,
For hate is the strongest of all emotions.

Searching For Daylight

20th November 1984 – 01:18

Feelings

My feelings lie frozen beneath the surface,
Like a blade of grass on a winter's day.
Still there, but unseen, unnoticed,
Frozen, safely packed away.
I smile and laugh, but cry inside deep down.
No one can see the darkness, there's nothing to
show,
But my mind is tortured, fearful
And the sadness just won't go.

Kathryn Shaw

27th November 1984 – 18:38

Intruder

I look at her, she turns away.
I talk to her, she does not hear.
She doesn't care, not about me,
I'm just a person who doesn't exist.
I see them talking, I turn away,
Pretend not to care, but I do,
Deep down inside a searing pain stabs,
And I don't know what to do.
I can't get through, she doesn't listen,
And it hurts more than anything,
Knowing it should be me she loves,
Instead of that intruder who takes my place

Searching For Daylight

29th November 1984 – 23:58

Visions

Life is a living vision,
People see what they want to see,
Just an image on the surface,
Of what they want life to be.
People don't want to delve deep down,
They just don't seem to care,
They are afraid of seeing
What life has hidden down there.
For underneath it's rotting,
Decaying from years of misuse,
Of people ignoring, not caring about
The years of ill abuse.
But time is getting longer,
And reality drifts away,
As the vision grows much stronger,
And life slowly ebbs away.

.3rd December 1984 – 18:28

Machines

Life is a long conveyor belt,
Carrying you to the end.
You flow in a line of many,
Treated the same in one long trend.
"Place one foot in front of the other",
In the beginning you learn to walk,
"Move your mouth communicate",
Just a formality, how to talk.
Pass through school and learn your lines,
Take exams, "you cannot fail!"
Wear a uniform, obey the rules,
Troop through classrooms in one long trail.
Out of school and more exams,
Find a job and earn your keep,
Jobs are scarce but life continues,
"In the day you work, at night you sleep".
No one must step out of line,
It's a sin to even try,
Keep all your feelings to yourself,
Laugh sometimes maybe but never cry.
Marry someone, reproduce,
Bring up your children well,
And then retire, prepare to die,
And go to heaven or hell.

Searching For Daylight

26th December 1984 – 13:37

Ambition

The aim, the point where have they gone?
Without them what is life?
Deflated, lost, there's no point living,
Without the strength of an ambition.
No mountain, towering, ready to climb,
No stretching bridge to cross
Nothing to do, no reason to live,
Everything has changed, all is lost.

6th January 1985 – 01:01

Time

Time ticks on, endless, infinite,
Always passing day by day,
A mysterious wheel, ever turning,
Sweeping people on their way.
Another year gone, more ahead,
A stretching sea of time.
A life of lies and fear and hatred,
Ending with one death-bringing chime.

Searching For Daylight

15th January 1985 – 18:12

Daybreak

Dawn is breaking, eyes are opening,
Slowly flickering as day begins.
The air is frozen, frosting eyelids,
That slowly open to welcome light.

My slow tread brings icy crunches,
From the sheet of snow that lies about.
Streets deserted in winter coldness,
Everyone's warm, I'm cold alone.

The solitude, though numb, is welcome,
Thoughts come easy in empty space.
Day's bustling confusion is way ahead of me,
The mind needs to clear when thinking of life
.
Lights in houses flash on around me,
As people get up to begin a new day,
Everyone's life is a new separate pathway,
They cross, or twist, or go on alone.

Mine is alone and stretches for ever,
Seemingly straight, though twisted inside.
It is where I am heading that fills my mind,
My frozen pathway, where will it end?

Kathryn Shaw

18th January 1985 – 22:14

Watching and Waiting
Sit and watch the world go by,
All the people as they pass,
Moving slowly here and there,
Visions drifting behind the glass.

Sit and watch out of your window,
See all the hate and every lie.
Watch all the fear, deceit, destruction,
Just sit and look and stare and sigh.

Watch all the men killing each other,
For any reason they might see.
Destroy for love of religion or country,
It's not the way the world should be.

Searching For Daylight

20th January 1985 – 18:46

Crying Inside

Frosty feelings below the surface,
Weeping with sadness, bitter with hate.
Restricted from movement, frozen in silence,
Nothing to do but shiver and wait.
Teardrops stinging behind closed eyelids,
Secreted from a mind too confused to explain,
But life goes on and I must live it,
Often wishing I could begin again.
Words won't explain how I feel right now,
I don't think I even really know.
The only thing I have left to do,
Is just hope and wish these feelings will go.
For slowly they are destroying me,
The thoughts inside the depths of my mind.
I daren't start searching for what is left there,
For I'm so unsure and scared what I'll find.

22nd January 1985 – 01:24

Winter

Snow lies frozen on clotheless trees,
As they stand slowly shivering,
In the bitter-frost icyness
Of the sharply-cold winter breeze.
The land around is white and dead.
Smothered in winter's cold blanket,
Sending the land and trees to sleep,
In dreams branches droop, heavy as lead.

Searching For Daylight

22nd January 1985 – 20:04

Headlights

Headlights shining, searching, waiting,
Trying to find the hidden way,
Through the dark damp mists of sadness,
Looking for the light of day.
Sadness settles, rotting, killing,
No chink of light is left still bright,
Mists roll in, hindering eyesight,
Light to darkness, day to night.
Cobwebs form in rotting corners,
The mind's in stages of decay,
You try so hard to break the gloom,
But hate steps out and blocks your way.
And slowly, sadly, light grows weaker,
Headlights dimming, flickering, gone!
And dark triumphant closes over,
Hooded, evil, hate has won.

Kathryn Shaw

17th February 1985 – 00:24

The Unknown Soldier

No one cares for the unknown soldier
Who lies, slowly dying, in the wounded ward.
Staring into memories distant,
Lost in the past, still back in the war.
His head is filled with the sound of gunshots,
His mind still fighting a lonely battle.
He lies back staring, but seeing what?
Not a whitewashed ward, but a blood-filled field.
He shakes every time he hears a plane,
Re-living his terror of times far gone.
Yet when someone speaks he hears nothing,
Or does he hear, and just not respond?
Maybe he's waiting this unknown soldier,
Waiting for his life to slip away.
Maybe he sees no point in living,
With the world as it is still fighting its wars.
And who can blame him, the unknown soldier,
With war-scarred body and distant eyes.
For why should he live, when the country he loved,
Took no notice of his feelings
And sent him out to die?

Searching For Daylight

24th April 1985 – 23:37

The Storm

Storms come suddenly, blocking the light,
The sun disappears from view,
And all around a darkness falls,
A midnight cloak sweeps over the land.

Storm-filled clouds threaten from above,
Mumbling angrily in the sky,
They loom dark and menacing as death,
Then slowly, sadly, begin to cry.

Then faster – torrents streaking down,
Soaking, saturating everywhere,
Rushing streams carry dying life,
'Til all the land is dead and bare.

Then suddenly they disappear,
The clouds, retreating, lift away,
Warmth, returning, steams the land,
And night surrenders to the heat of day.

But the storm, attacking's done its task,
The warmth cannot form life from death,
The earth is crumbling, foundations gone,
And looking around, there's nothing left.

Kathryn Shaw

27th April 1985 – 23:57

Valley of Despair

The valley of despair is a lonely place,
Far beyond dreams in a distant land.
You get there by sinking so low in your mind,
That you slip and fall, far down below.

The sides are so steep and the rocks so heavy,
That once you're there, there's no escape.
There's no one there to reach out and help you
And no company than that of your mind.

It's constantly night and the rain falls steadily,
Until every last feeling you have is gone.
You forget before, when the days were light,
When you could smile and the sun always shone.

You're stuck for all time in a living nightmare,
With the whisper of wind in the far away trees.
Nothing to do but lie down in the rubble
And be carried away by the lonely breeze.

Searching For Daylight

June 1985

Contradictions

Walking through a forest without any trees,

Being carried by the wind, when there isn't any breeze,

Telling endless truthful stories, when every one's a lie.

Tears streaming, falling, but I don't know how to cry.

A beautiful picture mounted in an empty frame.

Rows of different people, but every one's the same,

Shivering from the cold when the sun is beating down,

Swimming strongly, swiftly, but still having to drown.

Because the world is full of sadness

And the world is full of hate,

And however light your mind may feel,

You're dragged down by its weight.

5th July 1985 – 23:15

Sleep

Sleeping is an escape through misty dreams,
A world of fantasy and freedom.
The mind can drift wherever it wishes,
Laws and restrictions do not exist.

Hopelessness forgotten and left behind
In the cruel world of harsh reality,
Where despair filled people struggle on,
Trying to make sense of a life of lies.

Dreaming breaks all the invisible chains
And the floating, fleeing mind is free,
To wander into clouds of happiness
And glowing visions of warm content.

But all that dreaming brings is visions,
Desperate attempts of the mind to escape,
But once the vision and dream are over,
The mind's thrown back to cold reality.

The long day must yet again be suffered,
Before the pains can be forgotten,
And the mind slips away into dreams,
That the body only knows are not real.

Searching For Daylight

26th September 1985 – 23:36

Fighting

If you have to stretch up high,
Just to try to reach the ground
And all around is darkness,
Filling you with trembling fear.

If the swirling, stormy seas
Are always above your head.
You feel you're always drowning,
With the land too far away.

Open up your bleary eyes,
Don't be too afraid to see.
If you do not look around,
You will never find your desire.

Stretch out with your weary arms,
Swim and fight the angry waves.
The sea will soon be calmer,
Land is never far away.

Keep on fighting, hoping, believing,
Dreams can and do come true.
Eventually the day will come
When the two doves meet in the willow.

October 1985

Insecurity

The sword of insecurity
Stabs and delves deeper than any.
Inflicting searing, painful wounds,
Cutting through feelings and thoughts.
The wound inflicted by the sword
Bleeds afresh with every new sorrow.
There are no scars to show on the outside,
But tears show the pain that is caused,
As the sword twists even deeper
And a little more hope is destroyed.

Searching For Daylight

November 1985

Illusion

The sun shines and penetrates
A misty veil of beauty.
Drooping flowers lift their heads
To absorb the rays of life.

Above them leap light-footed children,
Playing with laughter in their eyes.
Sunshine envelops small faces
And brightens them into smiles.

This world, my world, is a picture
Of beauty and confident love.
Nothing can steal it or harm it,
For what could does not now exist.

There is no more fear round the corner,
I can now approach anything,
With a fortitude as certain
As the warmth of the sun above.

But wait! The sky is clouding now.
My confidence! My certainty!
Darkness closes, the veil is lifted
And I wake from yet another dream.

Kathryn Shaw

PART 2

2004 – 2007

Aged 34 – 37

Searching For Daylight

21st July 2004

Letting Go

I don't want to be drowning,
I want to keep swimming.
I don't want to keep losing,
I want to be winning.
But time moves on and the clouds aren't lifting,
The bomb is still there, endlessly ticking.
Time's meant to heal but the waiting is hurting,
The pain is increasing and the healing's not
working.
I try to be strong – smiling and laughing,
But the acting is hard and it's all so tiring.
I can't keep the play going much longer,
But there aren't many options and I feel so weary.
At times the alternative seems so tempting,
An end to the pain, an escape from the torment.
At times I can hear my demons beckoning,
And it seems so right, much easier than existing.
They tell me those I left would be better without me,
And convince me at times it's the only real answer.
I push them away and open my eyes,
Consequences rush around and around in my
mind.
How could I leave those who love me so much,
And transfer to them all my pain and darkness.
But I'm growing weaker and the current feels
stronger,
And still some days, just drowning seems simpler.

Just letting go
And sinking…

August 2004

Innocence

Eyes wide, bright and shining
Pure happiness

Arms out, tightly cuddling
Pure love

Eyes closed, softly breathing
Pure peace

Children are our future
Protect them

The innocence of youth
So pure

Shield them from the terrors
Around us

For once the innocence
Is broken

It's gone, lost forever
Flown away

Searching For Daylight

7th November 2004

The Tree of Life

The tree stands, as it always has,
Alone, but proud, in its Majesty.
Old and gnarled, but yet still so strong.
Its endless mass of branches stretch forever.

On the end of one of the branches
A new, fresh green bud slowly uncurls
To reveal a beautiful new leaf,
Sparkling brightly along with so many more.

The soft dew blankets them in its midst,
They feed and grow with their innocence,
Stronger with every passing day,
To mature individuals amongst the crowd.

But, almost before they realise,
Spring and summer are just memories.
The warm sun replaced with a chill
Representing inevitable autumn.

They turn to such beautiful colours,
Ironically hiding the painful truth.
For the bright reds, gold and oranges
Mask the beginning, the onset, of death.

The morning dew is replaced with frost,
Encrusting each leaf with painful grip.
Slowly sucking the life from within,
As they wither, curl and fall to the ground.

Kathryn Shaw

The tree stands as it always has,
Alone, and saddened with its secrets.
Every year the cycle continues,
On and on into eternity.

As sure as leaves grow, they all must fall,
It is just a matter of when.
For the tree of life, inevitably,
Is also the tree of death.

Searching For Daylight

6th December 2004

Turmoil

I try not to think but the thoughts still come.
I should stay and fight but I have to run.
All my thoughts just overwhelm me.
My understanding has gone.
My mind won't stop, it's too confused.
I hate the coward I've become.
I've hurt all those who love me most.
They should not suffer my pain.
It's not them who've done everything wrong,
I know it's me who has to change.
I don't deserve another chance,
Though I know that I should try.
But how do I change the feelings
When they just make me want to cry?
How did it all come to this?
I know I've dug too deep.
Part of me wants to battle on
But the rest of me just wants to sleep.

19th December 2004

Nightmares

Fear looms threatening in the darkness,
Tightening its grip with every sharp breath.
Faces appear when least expected,
Every time you try to close your eyes.
Faceless faces are most frightening.
So close and yet not quite in focus.
Features blurred and yet still so clear.
Dark and menacing, always watching.
And now yet one more face has joined them.
How many more are there still waiting?
How much harm has already been done
By all those strangers on the sidelines?
I cannot help but lie and wonder
How many children are now in pain?
Maybe right at this very moment
By monsters in disguise let inside their lives.
Places that should be safe and friendly
Turn to prisons with no escape.
Nightmares turn into reality
And soon the two cannot be parted.
As time passes, so very slowly,
Defences are constructed, brick by brick.
Without realising their meaning,
These safeguards turn to prisons of their own.
But however tall and thick the walls are.
However safe you think you may be.
A simple fact is just forgotten,
Every prison has a door with a key.

Searching For Daylight

21st December 2004

Matt

Always a smile and so much to give,
Touching, brightening the darkest corners
That no-one else could seem to reach.
So many reasons for him to live.

Such a loss, such a waste you will say,
A special man, cut down in his prime,
Yet I'm sure he gave more in his short life
Than most people could ever dream to attain.

'Only the good die young' – no consolation
For family and friends left behind.
Yet you must believe there's a reason,
To help with your overwhelming grief,

And I'm sure that a spirit so bright,
Has been lifted gently by angels
To a place where his compassion
Can still lighten up the darkest of nights.

January 2005

Confusion

I don't want to sleep. I don't want to dream.
I don't want to lose control any more.
Sleep is an escape from reality
That in itself is too confusing to explain.

I just don't understand my mind any more
And I have to find the explanation,
But the road is confusing and painful
And I no longer trust my conclusions.

I feel as if I'm constantly fighting
But the enemy's obscured from vision,
So I don't know how to defend myself,
Or what it is that I'm fighting for.

I just don't know who I am any more,
And don't know what to expect of myself,
Only what others expect of me,
And I try so hard not to let them down.

I concentrate and commit to my work,
Acting the role that I know should be me.
Some part of logic must be left intact,
I smile on the surface and apply what must be.

I must not show the children my weakness.
Their innocence shouldn't suffer my pain.
The acting continues, my role just changes,
Playing the part that they want me to play.

Searching For Daylight

But the faces are there in the background,
Just waiting for me to lose control
So that they can infiltrate my nightmares,
And reach inside until they find my soul.

So I don't want to sleep and lose control,
Or is that now the answer I seek?
As a certain end to the pain I feel
Would be not to wake up from my sleep.

February 2005

Self-Hatred

The pressure inside is overwhelming,
Sometimes building up slowly over time.
Sometimes suddenly there, unbearable,
A physical pain in the depths of the mind.
There is only one way to release it,
And before I have time to realise,
I'm holding the answer in my hand,
Its blade glinting, almost hypnotic.
I press hard and cut as deep as I can,
And the pain is good so I cut again
As many times as I feel I need,
And the pain gets better as the wound grows
deeper.
Then suddenly realisation hits
And I watch the blood run down my arm.
Dripping in the sink, bright red on white,
But the feeling is still pleasurable.
My arm throbs with the pain inflicted,
But the pressure inside has eased from my mind.
The hate I feel has been appeased
And the pain I deserve is somehow now real.
But the release is only temporary,
Soon replaced with sadness and guilt.
I watch the blood dripping and question, why?
The answer's not found and I don't understand.
It just adds to the list of unanswered questions.
The endless circle going round and round,
And I feel the pressure building again,
One cycle ended and another one begins.

Searching For Daylight

28th February 2005

For Jamie

A new star twinkles in the sky.

Just one, amongst so many more,

Yet this one's special – yours alone

- A bond that no one else can share.

A new emotion has been born,

Its roots entwine your very soul.

Its shoots and buds will fill your hearts

With love you've never felt before.

4th March 2005

The End

The sun has stopped shining,
The birds have stopped singing.
My life has now ended
But should be beginning.

Dark shadows are falling
Where dawn should be breaking
And I just need to sleep
But cannot stop waking.

My body should be warm
But it won't stop shivering,
And my mind needs to rest
But it won't stop thinking.

I should feel compassion
But I can't stop hating,
And I should want to live
But death is still waiting,

And I know I should breath

But I'm suffocating.

Searching For Daylight

4th March 2005

Darkness

Dark thoughts, blacker than black,
Swirling round endlessly,
Reaching corners that I
Didn't know existed.

Fingers crawling, creeping,
Leaving behind a trail
Of blood, dripping, spreading
And all encompassing.

Black dreams, darker than dark,
So real, terrifying,
And overwhelming that
I can no longer breath.

I awake uncertain
Of my own consciousness,
And with a pain so real
That I question my mind.

Dark and black, black and dark.
There's only one answer.
Nothing else is real
And nothing else matters
Anymore
Except
Death.

Kathryn Shaw

11th March 2005

Self Destruction

Self Destruction – push the button
And watch me fall apart.
Inner turmoil, twisting, turning,
A knife inside my heart.

So much loathing, so much hatred,
Directed deep inside.
There's no words left, no excuses,
And nowhere left to hide.

The blade is sharp, cutting, stabbing,
I can't describe the pain.
My soul is lost, please forgive me,
I just cannot explain.

There's no way back, I've come too far,
The bridges washed away.
The coward inside me is too strong
To face another day.

Searching For Daylight

12th March 2005

Forgiveness

So much to forgive
So much to forget
Too much time to cry
Too much in my head
A long time has passed
In just one short breath
So much hurt's been done
Too many tears shed
What did I do wrong?
What did I do right?
Where is all my love?
Hope's obscured from sight
Tears fall softly down
For times long ago
Pain is in my heart
Only I can know
Hate is deep inside
My head hung in shame
So much I regret
No one else to blame

15th March 2005

Understanding

Day turns to dusk and dusk to dark
And shadows fade into the night.
A pale moon glows and draws the tide
And the countryside sighs and sleeps.

Soft clouds wander across the sky,
Gently, sleepily suspended
Upon the comfy feather bed
That is made by the wind's soft breath.

A myriad of jewels appear,
Twinkling magically above,
Stars from a million miles away,
That have long ago burnt and died.

My head rests back on cool green grass,
My eyes lit up with what I see
And calm surrounds my aching head,
As nature's beauty comforts me.

A warm hand extends to clasp mine
And suddenly I understand.
I should fear my dreams no longer,
My spirit guide accompanies me.

Searching For Daylight

8th April 2005

Highs and Lows

Emotions high, emotions low,
Turning, like the tide in a storm.
From happiness to deep despair,
Feelings fade but are then reborn.
Smiling, laughing, shaking, crying,
Change in just the blink of an eye.
One moment so strong and certain,
Then thoughts so black, you question, why?
And so the scales rise and fall,
Weakness weighs heavy on the mind
And hope is so light and so bright,
But just so much harder to find.
I pray for the day to arrive,
When joy will outweigh despair
And the darker moments retreat,
Until they are no longer there.
I wait for the day the tide turns,
Without washing my hope away,
And the driftwood left on the beach
Can dry in the warmth of the day.
Until then I cling to the good times
And try to avoid all the rain.
Turning my back on the dark clouds,
Until the sun can shine again.

14th April 2005

Strength

I was asleep but now I've woken,
My mind's now warm instead of frozen,
My heart had stopped but now it's beating,
I nearly died but now I'm breathing.
My thoughts, now clear, replace confusion,
My mind's still tired but it's still thinking,
The pain's not gone and I'm still hurting,
But hurting's good, it means I'm living.
I've taken blows that life has thrown me,
But turned away in case they hurt me,
Acknowledgement and realisation
Were just too much, so I ignored them,
Instead escaping from existence
Into internal hibernation,
A warm and somehow safe escape from
All things real, that could not touch me.
Pretence though could not last forever,
My attempt at self-preservation,
Although protecting those around me,
Could only lead to self-destruction.
I had to wake and look behind me,
Attempting just some comprehension,
Of how the blows have left me feeling,
And heal the scars that are still bleeding.
My awakening has led to hurting,
Not just for me but those I care for.
Guilt is still my own worst enemy,
The hate's still there so deep inside me,
But something's changed and made me stronger
And suddenly my feelings matter.

Searching For Daylight

I will no longer see them trodden
Into the dirt and left just rotting.
Its taken time but now I'm facing
Internal battles overwhelming.
I'm now awake, alive, still breathing,
But most important, now I'm fighting!

23rd April 2005

A Mother's Love

I watch him closely from a distance.
He's unaware of my attention,
So engrossed is he in childish play.
The love I feel is overwhelming.
Although his head's turned away from me,
I can picture his face so clearly.
Blue eyes dancing and sparkling with fun,
Features set in deep concentration.

His blonde curls dance in the gentle breeze,
Twinkling where drops of water nestle,
Curling into the nape of his neck,
Wild and free like his youthful passion.
I let myself float into his mind,
Allow myself to know his senses.
The scent of salt, sea and sun lotion
So deliciously intermingled.

Water splashing coolly on his legs,
Sand and shingle pressed between his toes,
The warm sun delightful on his back,
Comforting like the warmth of my arms.
Sounds of the sea on the rocks around,
So gently rising, lapping, falling.
The background noise of the beach and sky –
Laughter, playful screams, seagulls soaring.

Searching For Daylight

His fishing net must be twice his height,
Ungainly wielded into the sea.
Hopefully lifted, water dripping,
Its murky contents studied with care.
I touch his soul and know his pleasure,
And feel so gratefully reassured,
That he allows himself happiness,
After feeling so empty with grief.

I watch him from a distance, closely,
Wishing I could hold him one more time,
Smell him, feel him, breath him, comfort him,
Let him know just how much I need him.
I hear a voice from far behind me,
And painfully know what I must do.
I take one last, long, lingering look,
Then turn to leave him for the last time.

11th May 2005

Love

Love is ageless
No time barriers need be crossed

Love shines a light
When all your emotions are lost

Love is so real
When so many people are false

Love is so true
In this crazy world that is not

Love fights despair
And pushes it far, far away

Love is constant
Through dark nights as well as the day

So don't fight love
Embrace it arms open, eyes wide

Time matters not
For you have love there at your side

One hour of love
Can end the years of hurt and pain

One hour of love
Can restore all your faith again

Searching For Daylight

12th May 2005

Alive

Love has no boundaries, no bars, locks or keys.
So totally indiscriminative,
And hence, age, race, colour and religion
Become irrelevant and meaningless.

Love has no concept of time that passes.
It is not shy and arrives unannounced,
Leaving you breathless with its speed and power,
Fulfilling and overwhelming your heart.

Love has no conscience and hence has no guilt.
Comes to rest with anyone, anywhere,
Its arrival often unexpected,
It settles easily, without a care.

Love is alive, this must be understood.
So often overlooked and forgotten,
Nurturing and care can be neglected,
And as with all things that live, it can die.

Love's requirements are not complicated:
A little attention, trust and kindness,
Help it thrive, grow, blossom and be strong,
And the fruits of its harvest are boundless.

Love can cause pain by its sudden absence,
For pain and love so often intertwine.
But just a week of true love in your heart is
Worth a year of loneliness any time.

28th May 2005

Pressure

Smothered, breathless, suffocating,
Fighting in the darkness, gasping.

Falling like a stone and spinning,
Arms flailing, hopelessly grasping.

Sinking, drowning, body powerless,
Turbulent water surrounding.

Darkness closing, life is weaker,
All is nothing, encompassing.

Breathing deeply, gulping, drinking,
Air is sweet and satisfying.

Flying like a bird and soaring,
Arms outstretched like wings and gliding.

Swimming quickly, body slicing
Water's mirror, cracked with power.

Light is awesome, almost blinding,
Forces meet and pull me nearer.

Breathing slows and I surrender,
Relaxing to something stronger.
Good or bad it draws me closer
And, like a drug, drags me under.

Searching For Daylight

Dying, breathing, falling, flying.
Drowning, swimming, blind or seeing.
Far apart and yet so similar.
Something, nothing, loser, winner.

Complications all to simple.
Solutions to something complex.
Answers found and then forgotten.
Future seen but then forsaken.

Life is full but yet so empty,
Always waiting for fulfilment,
But something bright guides me forward
And its strength is overwhelming.

Watching and hating, punishing.

Seeing and loving, comforting.

Kathryn Shaw

1st July 2005

Eternity

The enormity of eternity
Is reflected in the stars,
Sparkling with energy,
As they light the way to infinity.

As your dreams merge into reality,
So your chosen path appears,
Mapped in the constellations,
Guiding the way to immortality.

Hopes are born to change into achievements
And as each one is conquered,
A star shines bright in the sky,
As nature's permanent badge of honour.

Each one seemingly insignificant,
Yet so clear in its presence,
Important to the answer,
Part of the solution to life's jigsaw.

The expanse of space is just breathtaking,
Amazing by its absence,
So full with its emptiness
And so beautiful in its solitude.

The deepest of nights still turns into dawn
And the daylight hides the truth,
As the sun shines from the sky,
Masking its three-dimensionality.

Searching For Daylight

The answer is an unknown entity,
Any searching is in vain.
Just trust in your convictions,
The darkness of night will show you the way.

Kathryn Shaw

15th July 2005

Dreams of Hope

Drifting and dreaming, escaping in sleep,
The mind rises up so light and so free.
Floating gently, cautiously exploring,
Reaching out to places of happiness.

The crisp crunch of frost on the fresh green grass,
In the pale half-light of a winter's dawn.
The sharp cold cut of the air in your lungs,
As you breath the damp scent of the morning.

The glowing golden warmth of a fireside,
With flickering flames dancing in the dark.
The embers take on a life of their own,
A companion who's there all through the night.

Kicking through leaves of orange, red and gold,
Scooping an armful and letting them fly.
Wood smoke permeating the autumn chill,
Drifting through trees that rustle as they blow.

Surrounded by green on a summer's day,
With meadow-sweet grass scenting the air.
Bright sun humidly warm on your body.
The sky so blue, overwhelming your soul.

The misty wetness of a spring rainfall,
As you stand dripping, arms stretched to the sky.
A tree absorbing the essence of life,
A life welcoming a reason to cry.

Searching For Daylight

Restlessly shifting, now leaving your dreams,
Falling and pulled back into consciousness.
The subconscious transition to waking,
Body stirring, eyes open to the light.

Half-memories of dreams are still in the mind,
To accompany thoughts throughout the day.
Eyes shine bright recollecting the beauty,
Recognising hope in reality

23rd August 2005

Face the Storm

Cry into the wind
And your tears will dry
Before they leave your eyes.

Scream into the thunder,
Your voice will be lost
And your pain absorbed.

Stretch out to the rain,
It will hide your tears
Should they start to fall.

Do not fear the dark,
Your soul is your guide,
Its light always shines.

Always seek the sun,
It is never far
And will warm your heart.

Rise above the clouds,
They have no substance,
Then your eyes will see.

Turn and face the storm,
Cling to the future,
Leave the past to die.

Searching For Daylight

23rd August 2005

The Lost Children

(Like Billy)

Faces blank with resignation
And so pale – so grey –
With shadows where their eyes should be.

Shoulders droop with hopelessness –
Leaning into silence,
With childish laughter far away.
Dejected
Lost

Hearing words from tongues that deserve
To be ripped from bleeding mouths.
Seeing hatred that burns
And contaminates
And spreads.

Any act of liveliness is shouted down
And crushed
And twisted
And scorned
And turned around
And directed at the heart.

Their eyes are not those of children,
They have seen too much.

Their minds are not those of children,
They have known too much.

They are no longer children,
Just empty shells that function.
Harbouring future addicts, murderers,
Thieves and abusers.

They do not stand a chance.
It makes me cry.
So very sad
But true...

Searching For Daylight

September 2005

Drowning and Flying

Black mirror, dark as dark,
Embrace me and drown my silence.
Drag me to your depths
And hold me in your comforting arms.

Dark mirror, black as black,
Grant me inevitable peace.
May my last breath
Rise to your surface and be gone.

Dark mirror, do not fear,
For in the morning, you will be
Sparkling silver-blue,
Reflecting the sun and the sky
And my soul will float up
To your surface and fly,

And my hatred gone, I will be free.

October 2005

Chasing the light

Part 1

I chase the light, but it evades me.
Not quite in reach – it slips away,
Until it is a pinpoint in the distance,
A star lighting another hemisphere.

I dodge the shadows but they engulf me.
They grip me with icy fingers and I fall
Into the black hole of my mind,
Searching for meaning in memories and dreams.

I surrender to the dark as it pulls me
And drags me spinning to its core,
Until I no longer care about the light.
If it appears I will turn away.

All has inverted, external becomes internal,
Clarity is lost in the confusion,
Understanding is buried for ever,
And the only hope left longs for the end.

Searching For Daylight

Part II

I close the door and turn the key,
My solitude is all I need.
I bar the windows, draw the blinds
And sit inside my prison mind.

The floor is hard, the room is cold,
The stale damp air is all I breath.
I sit and shiver in the dark,
I sit and cry where no-one sees.

For I have seen the end is near,
My eyes have seen their final dawn.
I know now this cannot be changed
And somehow this brings me relief.

I cannot mend the broken glass,
The pieces shattered all around.
I crush some tightly in my hand,
The blood feels good where it runs warm.

I close my eyes and look inside
And hate the pictures that I see.
But nothing's left to fight the storm
And nothing's left to turn the key.

Part III

I need to run but the door is locked,
And anyway, where would I go?
There is nowhere – just a black hole
Of ever increasing nothing.

Faces surround me full of anger –
I turn to see their target
And find myself looking in the mirror
That hangs on the door to my mind.
Hatred overwhelms me and I watch myself scream,
Over and over, wishing the pain were gone,
But it is part of me,
Embedded in my soul…

Afterwards, I watch myself lying
So still and peaceful,
Surrounded by flowers
And hypocritically mourning faces.

The pain has gone. It lies invisibly beside me.
The hatred has been appeased
And I watch myself smile,
As my soul rises up and is free.

Searching For Daylight

September 2006

Once Upon a Time

Dreams and fairytales, nightmares and reality.
Twisting and evil, the forest of thorns
Cannot be broken with enchanted swords.
The Handsome Prince is a fraud, using his charm
To lure innocent children to destruction.

'Happily ever after' belongs far away,
In fictitious memories, in long ago dreams.
In the place where the setting sun is lost,
As it sinks into the red ocean of clouds.

The wolves aren't real as they chase me through my sleep,
But fear distorts the difference and I cannot hide.
Fairytales are the root of children's nightmares,
As 'Once Upon a Time' turns into 'Never Again'.

I cannot breath, a dead weight presses my face
Into suffocation, and the darkness spins round and round.
I want it to stop, but know that waking will be worse,
With comprehension that the nightmare is real…

A young child with a stick draws pictures in the dirt –
Smiling faces, happy families – her mother calls
And she jumps up, runs to her, the wind in her hair,
Not seeing that as she turns away,
It blows the dust, and her dreams are gone.

October 2006

Peace and Candlelight

The pain flows like water down a waterfall,
Fast and furious, then sinking far below.
Torrents too fast and too deep to contain,
But all I want is peace and candlelight.

My angels call me and say 'hold on!'
They kiss my aching head and hold me
Above the flowing water that surrounds me,
But all I want is peace and candlelight.

Seconds flow too fast and become years
That should not seem so timeless,
But looking back nothing was right,
And all I want is peace and candlelight.

The time has all been wrong and change is futile.
Are they angels, or demons tempting me to more
pain?
Confusion surpasses reality, and I cry
That all I want is peace and candlelight.

The church is cool and dark and smells
Of the childhood that haunts my dreams.
I sit and watch, detached, watching but not being.
All I wanted was peace and candlelight.

Searching For Daylight

Tears stream down faces that I know but never knew,
And the flowers are already dying in the wreaths
That surround me, as I lie in my accomplishment.
I finally have peace and candlelight.

But what will be there when the candles have burnt?
That is a question unanswerable by the living,
But it cannot be worse than the pain of now,
And all I want is peace and candlelight
    - Then darkness!

October 2006

The Cycle of Life

The fine line between life and death is translucent
As the horizon of the heavy autumn sky,
Where it meets the furthest view of the deep grey
sea.

The cycle completed, as mother reverts to
newborn,
And the daughter becomes the parent, as she
gently strokes
The fragile cheek, with finger touch as soft as a
feather.

The last gasps of breath are frantic and desperate
As those first gulps of air from a baby at birth.
The fear in staring eyes is as in a mirror.

It is the unknown that is in the reflection,
Clearly seen in the open windows to the soul.
The fear of death as certain as the fear of life.

Until finally, the look of fear is replaced by peace.
For angels gentle wings encompass the soul of the
dead,
As surely as a mother's arms enfold her newborn
child.

For as a baby is surrounded by the natural love
Of her family of the future, the soul of the deceased
Is greeted and encompassed by her loved ones of
the past.

Searching For Daylight

It is this realisation that brings the look of peacefulness
To the faces of old and new, as, on either side of the line,
They leave this world as they enter, close in their hearts to those they love.

Kathryn Shaw

October 2006

The Unborn Child

The sun glows red and sinks in the sky,
Into the tide of clouds below.
Somewhere a dead leaf drifts and blows,
Like a bird from a golden cage of long ago.

The cage-lock breaks and a baby falls
Down from the skies, cradle and all,
Like the nursery rhyme from the childhood it will not
know.

The cradle's a basket woven of reeds,
It lands in a stream and like Moses of the past,
The baby of the future floats and cries.
Cries that cut your soul for the past it does not
know
And for the future that it somehow perceives.

The stream flows on into the river,
Its colours changing as they always do –
From silver to black, from black to gold,
But finally reaching the blood-red sea

The cries cease, the child stretches its arms to the
angels,

Meets the setting sun, takes one last breath, dies,
and is gone.

74

Searching For Daylight

October 2006

Regrets and Retribution

If I could turn back time,
I would undo what has been done.
I would make sure that your eyes
Had opened to the sun.

I would hold you so close,
Our hearts would beat as one.
I'd kiss your tiny lips,
So gentle and so warm.

The pain I feel inside
Is tearing me apart.
I took your life away,
Destroyed your beating heart.

Your perfect soul was lost,
Before it had begun.
Your spirit, I've destroyed,
I search for where it's gone.

The hate I feel inside
Is more than I can take.
I don't deserve to live.
A soul for a soul.
A life for a life.
I didn't know black
 Could be
 So black.
I'm sorry.

January 2007

Angels and Vultures

All is reversed and the clock ticks backwards,
Symmetry is lost in the confusion of the transition.
Shapes are no longer three-dimensional – they turn
Flat, as feelings revert to that of a child.

Right is as wrong as all the choices ever made,
And chances that should have been taken are lost
In the shadows of the future, as it is consumed by
the
Past, that overwhelms and overturns the present.

The sun rises in the West and sets in the East, and
Its blood-red shadows run in rivers into the night.
The dawn is greeted by the setting sun, by the
Clouds drifting across the moon, as it is pulled by
the tide.

Gravity drags me upwards, towards the blazing
sun,
And my tears fly away and turn to steam, as
My body is burnt, and then freezes in the coldness
Of the sun, as its rays turn to ice like my heart.

Presents opened in excitement are empty boxes
That make the children cry, as anticipation
becomes
As dead as the bodies beneath gravestones, and
they
Realise that life is only a means to certain death.

Searching For Daylight

The lost children turn to Angels, and circle around
Like Vultures awaiting the next victim of the
Celebration that will be theirs, when the next lucky soul
Takes their last breath, and can finally be free.

But worse are the souls of the Unborn, for they are
Trapped in the darkness between sunset and sunrise.
They do not even know enough to feel hatred.
They will never be Angels or Vultures,
Just Shadows
That might have been.

www.ingramcontent.com/pod-product-compliance
Lightning Source LLC
Chambersburg PA
CBHW031220290326
41931CB00035B/623